Sleep Paralysis

Learn How to Stop Sleep Paralysis and What Causes It to Begin with

by Carter Andersen

Table of Contents

Introduction 1

Chapter 1: An Overview of Sleep Paralysis............................ 7

Chapter 2: The Actual Experience of Sleep Paralysis 11

Chapter 3: How to Manage an Episode Calmly 15

Chapter 4: Effectively Treating Sleep Paralysis 19

Chapter 5: Using an Episode to Your Advantage.................. 23

Conclusion.. 27

Introduction

One scenario: You are beginning to wake up from a dream. You are on your back, but realize that you can't move. You try and try again, but you still have problems moving. Your eyes remain closed and you have problems opening them as well. It feels like someone is holding you down, and your heart begins to beat fast because you don't know what is really going on. After about 3 minutes, (which in reality was actually 5 seconds) you are broken from your chains and your eyes pop open.

Another scenario: You are in the middle of a dream and you are quite enjoying it. Then all of a sudden everything turns dark and it feels as though death is approaching. What's happening? You start panicking, screaming even, and wake up in terror. You've just woken your spouse up and even your dog downstairs. They wonder what has happened, but you have no idea.

Last scenario: you go to bed one night, after a long day at work. The only thing on your mind is to put your eye mask on and drift to dreamland. You lie down, and feel yourself drifting to sleep. But right before you lose consciousness, you feel your 'soul' being dragged down through the bed, through the ground, and maybe even to the pits of hell. You go into a panic and wake up, feeling your heartbeat race and your breaths short and quick. What has just happened? Why did it feel like dying, you ask yourself?

These three scenarios may sound like something straight from a Halloween special. But horror stories like these are experiences many people really suffer from at night. Some have only felt this type of thing once in their life, while others experience these nightmarish scenarios often. This phenomenon is referred to as "sleep paralysis", which occurs when a person is unable to move or react either as he falls asleep or upon waking up. The three scenarios listed above for some people are only the tip of the iceberg, where they continue to hallucinate and experience visions of ghosts and other apparitions. This is why sleep paralysis has caused many folklore and legends to pop up throughout the millennia. Nowadays, many scientists believe that many of the stories people tell about ghosts and alien abductions have come about as a result of sleep paralysis.

There is no specific drug to help remedy this condition. It is further impossible to predict its next occurrence in order to stop it. What can be done, however, is to change our sleeping habits and other facets of our lifestyle in an attempt to control and mitigate it. In addition, some people are more predisposed to sleep paralysis than others. If you have a history of panic attacks, then chances are that you will suffer sleep paralysis episodes at one time or another. In this book, we'll discuss sleep paralysis in greater detail, including what really causes it, why it happens to us, and what we can do to manage and prevent it. If you're ready to learn more, let's get started!

3

© Copyright 2015 by Miafn LLC - All rights reserved.

This document is geared towards providing reliable information in regards to the topic and issue covered. The publication is sold with the idea that the publisher is not required to render accounting, officially permitted, or otherwise, qualified services. If advice is necessary, legal or professional, a practiced individual in the profession should be ordered.

- From a Declaration of Principles which was accepted and approved equally by a Committee of the American Bar Association and a Committee of Publishers and Associations.

In no way is it legal to reproduce, duplicate, or transmit any part of this document in either electronic means or in printed format. Recording of this publication is strictly prohibited and any storage of this document is not allowed unless with written permission from the publisher. All rights reserved.

The information provided herein is stated to be truthful and consistent, in that any liability, in terms of inattention or otherwise, by any usage or abuse of any policies, processes, or directions contained within is solely and completely the responsibility of the recipient reader. Under no circumstances will any legal responsibility or blame be held against the publisher for any reparation, damages, or monetary loss due to the information herein, either directly or indirectly.

Respective authors own all copyrights not held by the publisher.

The information herein is offered for informational purposes solely, and is universal as so. The presentation of the information is without contract or any type of guarantee assurance.

The trademarks that are used are without any consent, and the publication of the trademark is without permission or backing by the trademark owner. All trademarks and brands within this book are for clarifying purposes only and are the owned by the owners themselves, not affiliated with this document.

Chapter 1: An Overview of Sleep Paralysis

To understand how you can properly manage sleep paralysis, you must first understand what sleep paralysis really is. Actually, sleep paralysis is still not fully understood by experts either, but we are able to recognize why people experience many things featured in horror films. Let's look at history first – sleep paralysis throughout the ages.

Sleep paralysis is a fairly new term, and the actual workings behind the phenomenon remained unknown for many until the last century. Before this, different cultures around the world came up with their own superstitious ideas to try and explain what was happening. It was Samuel Johnson who coined the term 'nightmare,' which describes most of the symptoms of sleep paralysis. In the past, people interpreted not being able to move during the night to be a demon lying on their chest. Europeans called these "demons" mares, so basically the word nightmare translates to 'night demon.' Different cultures have their own interpretations of the mare, as well as their own idea regarding its appearance and behavior.

In Scandinavian folklore for example, the mare looks like a woman, not a Victoria's Secret model, but rather a very ugly woman controlled by supernatural forces. This woman visits all the homes in the village and lies on the inhabitants' chests, causing them to experience the symptoms of sleep paralysis accompanied by bad dreams. Pointing to far away countries is hardly necessary as the southern states have their own versions of the mare. They refer to the mare as the 'witch riding.' Phrases like "the witch is riding you" or "the haint is riding you" might sound familiar if you are from one of the southern states.

The unnerving thing about sleep paralysis for many people is that it is brought on by supernatural beings. Many people grow up to believe that demons are responsible for feeling constrained at nights, and start visiting their pastor more often to get a clearer picture as to why the devil is bothering them so much. If you have experienced seeing heavenly (or otherworldly) bodies floating across your room shortly after waking up, if you feel symptoms of terror and panic, and you are not free to move, then you are experiencing sleep paralysis. Sleep paralysis happens when you wake up out of REM (rapid eye movement) sleep. Now, most people have heard about REM, but are not sure what it really is. REM is basically the period of sleep where you are in your deepest sleep. This is where most of your dreams take place, especially the ones you reminisce about when you wake up in the morning. It's called REM sleep because your eyes move around very fast, and your breath is spaced and very slow. However, the muscles in your body are on lockdown, and you are actually, by the true definition of the word, paralyzed. So why would the brain and your body do this? Isn't paralysis bad? Actually, paralysis in REM sleep is very good. If your muscles aren't on lockdown, then chances are you will act out your dreams. Surely you don't want to be able to jump off a rooftop and fly in your dreams and be fearful that you might be doing that in real life. Thanks to different neurotransmitters in the brain, the body is safe from hurting itself and others during the deepest stages of sleep.

9

10

Chapter 2: The Actual Experience of Sleep Paralysis

During a sleep paralysis episode, your mind suddenly wakes up from an REM dream, but your body is still asleep. The panic first sets in when a person realizes that they can't move or speak, in addition to not being able to breathe sometimes or experiencing hallucinations. When suffering this phenomenon after just having woken up, sometimes a person will feel like their breath is being sucked out of their chest. Turkish folklore has an explanation for this symptom which they call the 'karaban', or 'the dark presser.' This creature goes into people's rooms at night, pressing on their chest, while stealing their breath. Why would this creature do such a thing? No one knows.

It is really refreshing to know that science has a great explanation for this phenomenon. Can you imagine something being done to your body by an outside force and you can't control or stop it? The very thought is pretty frightening. People don't experience sleep paralysis the same way. While some may see demons floating over their chest, others will feel themselves floating off to the cosmos, and yet others will feel like they're dying. Some may experience it for just a fraction of a second, others a second or two, and some will experience sleep paralysis for as long as several minutes. Studies have shown that for a person with supernatural beliefs or who might feel as though death is approaching, experiencing these symptoms can be very distressing. The findings show that the more a person is educated about the condition, the less likely they are to be distressed about it. Hence, the best way to fight this condition is to better acquaint yourself with it and the reason why your body is experiencing it. So let's recap the most common symptoms of this condition:

- Fear
- Confusion
- Inability to move the limbs
- Trouble breathing and/or a heavy chest
- Feeling of doom and sudden death
- Visual and auditory hallucinations

Sleep paralysis is not a disease. So it is hardly necessary to go rushing to your doctor if you experience it. Chances are that most people will experience a symptom of sleep paralysis at least once in their lifetime. Some, unfortunately, suffer from a disorder which causes the experience to become more frequent. It can be very annoying, and sometimes scary.

Even though you don't have to rush to the doctor if you are experiencing the abovementioned problems, chances are that you could be experiencing these problems based on a more serious condition than sleep paralysis or sleep paralysis disorder alone. One of these conditions is narcolepsy. Narcolepsy is a neurological disorder that occurs when a person is unable to distinguish between being asleep and awake normally. Narcoleptic people feel an excessive need to sleep during the daytime, and will often find their sleep disturbed during the night time. A normal person experiences REM sleep in about an hour or two after falling asleep, while narcoleptics experience REM during the first 5 minutes of sleep. Narcoleptics sometimes experience cataplexy, which is an episode of muscle weakness, ranging from mild to severe, or a sudden burst of consciousness, where they are surprised, happy, angry or fearful at what has just happened. It can occur during the day or nighttime, and is a form of sleep paralysis. Narcoleptics experience the other symptoms of sleep paralysis, such as hallucinations, as they fall asleep during these episodes.

Other conditions that could cause sleep paralysis are migraines, anxiety disorders and sleep apnea. If you think you are narcoleptic, you should definitely see a doctor. If you experience any other symptoms, and they start to worry you, you should see your doctor. Your doctor can make a proper diagnosis to see if there is any underlying factor behind your sleep paralysis episodes. Once you know what is going on, then you can take steps in either managing your episodes or treating them.

Chapter 3: How to Manage an Episode Calmly

You can manage your episodes easily. If you experience them often, the trick is to be aware of what you are going through, and what can be done to manage it. You will then be able to control the way your body feels, and you can also snap yourself out of it.

When experiencing an episode, where you are unable to move after just waking up, the trick is to focus on your body. Not your whole body, but just a part of your body. Remember, paralysis occurs mainly in the arms, the legs, the chest, the abdomen and the throat. You may not be able to move your limbs, but what you can do to wake yourself up is to move a single body part like your toe or your finger. Just keep wagging and moving these body parts until you wake up. You may have heard of wiggling your toes to wake up out of a dream. It works brilliantly during sleep paralysis as well. Keep wiggling your toe or your finger and the paralysis will cease. Even moving your tongue will help. You can also try clenching and unclenching your fists as well.

Focus on the movement of your eyes. Even when dreaming you are awake but you really are not, you can wake up by moving your eyes around. Moving your eyes back and forth will help break the paralyzed state and doing it as fast as possible will break your paralysis straight away.

15

The next thing you should do is to not fight with what is happening. You are experiencing a symptom of paralysis so deal with it, don't fight it. Not only does fighting not help, since fighting involves struggling to move your arms and other major limbs, but it also puts you into a state of panic and intensifies it. The trick is to learn to go with the flow, accept what is happening, and breathe. Relax and surrender when you feel this happening to you during your sleep. Sure it feels strange, and sure the feeling of levitation and dying is not pretty, but you have to go with the flow in order for you to break out of it without waking up in a panic. Relax the moment you feel it happening to you, and then focus on your breathing. Controlling the intake of breaths has been taught for millennia as an excellent relaxation tactic, and breath control will help you relax during a sleep paralysis episode. It is not enough to just do this when you are sleeping. You should practice your breathing when you are awake too! During the day, at odd hours, practice taking in deep and slow breaths, then letting out the air slowly. When you control your breathing during one of your episodes, it will help you relieve some of the tightness and pains in your chest that you may be experiencing. You heart will be beating fast during these episodes, and controlled breathing will help bring your heart to a steady rate and rhythm again. It can't be stressed enough how important breathing is during these episodes, as people suffering from sleep paralysis often forget to breathe. Once you've controlled your breathing, then your body will force itself to wake up.

Finally, you can manage your sleep paralysis episodes by letting your loved one know what happens to you at night, and how they can help. If you talk to your partner, describing the symptoms you experience during such times, they will know what to look for in such moments. For instance when they notice a shortness of breath in you or see that you are struggling to get awake, they are prepared to help you. They will know how to do it in a way that will not harm you. Hence, rapid and vigorous shaking is a no-no. Also, talk to your partner about your beliefs as well as his or hers, and how your beliefs may affect how you experience your sleep paralysis episodes. The name of the game is understanding, and it is only through understanding and knowledge that you will truly be able to conquer this annoying condition.

Chapter 4: Effectively Treating Sleep Paralysis

Why manage your sleep paralysis when often times we can prevent it. Treatment methods are not 100% effective, and chances are there will be times that you will experience symptoms even when following everything to the letter. But once you follow the very few steps in treating and preventing sleep paralysis, you will have a much better sleeping experience. It must also be noted that there is no drug that treats sleep paralysis on its own, unless the sleep paralysis is being brought on by another medical condition such as narcolepsy and migraines, in which case, medication treatment is prescribed and given by a doctor.

The group of people that seems to be most affected by this condition are either sleep deprived people, or people with truly disturbed sleep patterns. In these cases, the best way to deal with sleep paralysis is to sleep. And not only to sleep, but to have a proper sleep schedule where the body is away from sunlight for at least 6 hours. This is how nature intended it, so going to bed at 5 am on weekends isn't helping at all. Therefore, the best way to treat your condition is to develop a good sleeping schedule that works great for you. Sure it is hard, especially for busy working people who have late night meetings and assignments, but for your own health and sanity you should try your best to ensure that you maintain a proper sleeping pattern. Also, if you have a habit of drinking caffeinated drinks and beverages or alcohol before you go to bed, stop doing it, as you have a good chance of inducing a sleep paralysis episode. If you cannot get the recommended 7-8 hours of sleep each night, make sure you get some naps during the day time. Napping will help you make up for lost sleep time, and will also help you get even more focused for the rest of the day's tasks.

When in bed, ensure that you sleep on your sides. It is a very uncomfortable thing to do for people who don't usually do this, since we all have our preferred sleeping positions, but you will get the hang of it soon enough and it may very well become your favorite sleeping position in the future. As you may notice, most of the sleep paralysis attacks happen when you are on your back. You do not suddenly become immune to these attacks when you lie on your side, however. Plus, you roll around during the night, so you should place safeguards on your nightwear, such as a blunt object at the back of your shirt to prevent you from staying on your back.

The best things to prevent sleep paralysis episodes from happening can be practiced during daytime. These things include exercise and eating. It is important to exercise regularly, and also eat the right foods. Identify any trigger that may be causing your episodes. These triggers could be a medication, or a certain food that you have been eating. Ensure that you avoid these substances like the plague, and replace them if possible.

Finally, see your doctor. Do not panic, as your sleep paralysis is not a disease. It is just an annoying condition, but if you experience it more than once per month, it could either mean you have a sleep paralysis disorder, or you have other underlying factors that are a bit more serious, such as narcolepsy. In these cases, your doctor will thoroughly examine you by looking at your medical history, and listening to all your previous experiences. They will then advise you what your next course of action should be.

Chapter 5: Using an Episode to Your Advantage

For some, sleep paralysis is a very scary experience. For others it's just an annoying experience they wish they could get rid of. Some learn to live with it, while some allow the conditions to keep them up at night. Some are affected by the disorder on a regular basis, while some are afflicted by it just once or twice in their lives. Those who experience it on a regular basis have sleeping paralysis disorder. This is when they experience the condition more than once in a month. If you have experienced sleep paralysis on a regular basis, then it's time to use it to your advantage. However, attempt this only if you have an open mind and an adventurous spirit. So, if you're not one of these people, you could either skip this chapter or, if you're curious enough, continue reading.

The number one thing to oversee when taking control of your sleep paralysis episodes is your fear. You cannot take charge if you are fearful of it. How can you control a horse if you are scared of it? How can you control your child if you are scared of him? Building enough courage to know what you are facing and what you are about to face is important in controlling your sleep paralysis. So every time you experience a sleep paralysis episode, whether it involves seeing a hallucination or feeling like you're about to die, it is important to calm your nerves. It is important to get rid of the fear of the unknown, and what better unknown is there than death itself. There's a chance that you will feel shortness of breath and a heavy heartbeat rate. The trick is to breathe slowly and breathe deeply.

Now the second thing to know when trying to take control of your sleep paralysis is how to differentiate fiction from reality. This is called lucid dreaming, where you are able to know when you are dreaming, and know how to control your dreams and be in charge of your actions. It's a common theme in our dreams to feel helpless of what happens in them. Whether it be a dream about us getting run down by a scary clown, or being beaten up by a school bully, or falling from the sky, or going to work without our pants on, only a few of us have truly mastered how to prevent those dreams from happening, or to control them by making those situations turn to our favor. Lucid dreaming is an art, and it will take some practice. The art of lucid dreaming is scary to some, while for others it is immoral as well. However, not being able to take charge of your actions in your dreams sucks, and there's absolutely nothing worse than having those dreams become nightmares. During your sleep paralysis episode, if your eyes are open and you're hallucinating, remember to breathe in slowly and calm yourself, then close your eyes and imagine how you want your situation to be. Some people experience this part with their eyes closed – a dream inside a dream is what they call it. This is where you believe you are awake because you see your room, but in actuality, you're not able to move, and you might see some scary beings around you and have a feeling of doom. The room seems so real because that's the way you saw the room before you fell asleep, or that's the way you've seen the room in the past when waking up. Just remember to follow the procedure - close your eyes and know you're not awake. In these types of dreams you may realize that you're not awake, and try to wake yourself up. You then realize that you can't, and start panicking until you finally wake up. As said earlier, the trick is to put yourself in a happier place, a place you feel you can control. Don't panic, relax. You're actually putting yourself back to sleep, and entering dreamland again, but this time you are in control of what is happening.

So, think really hard that you are flying over a field of dandelions, for instance. Close your eyes, relax, and enter your very own wonderland. Keep focus on your thoughts, and it will become reality. It's important to maintain practice, because if you lose focus, you will either wake up or slip into a nightmare. After this, the final thing to do is just to go with the flow. It will feel weird at first, and it might be short-lived the first time you do it, but once you've done it, it will be a rewarding experience. You can use these techniques not only to induce lucid dreaming during periods of sleep paralysis, but you will also be able to do it any time you want.

Conclusion

Sleep paralysis is a frightening experience many have experienced at least once in their lifetime. Some people experience it on a regular basis, and it can be very frustrating at times. If you're one of these people, just know that it gets better once you change the right things. Sometimes sleep paralysis can be attributed to more than one factor, so despite trying the suggested methods you still experience it from time to time. In these cases, you can just teach yourself to ignore the symptoms. Some people have lived with this condition for years, still they get all the sleep they need and are happy throughout the day. All it takes is to remind yourself that what you are experiencing is not actual death trying to creep up on you, but just an anomaly of the nervous system. Every time you experience any of these symptoms in the night, you may jerk awake, but just take a deep breath, think happy thoughts and go back to sleep. Also, make sure that you stick to a good sleeping schedule.

Sleep paralysis just loves to ride on a person who goes to bed whenever they feel like, even if it's 5 in the morning. Getting a good night's rest is important in making sure you don't experience these symptoms too regularly. Plus, if you're adventurous and curious enough, you could use it to your advantage. Let tonight be the last night sleep paralysis troubles you.

Finally, I'd like to thank you for purchasing this book! If you found it helpful, I'd greatly appreciate it if you'd take a moment to leave a review on Amazon. Thank you!

Printed in Great Britain
by Amazon